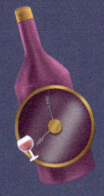

Why It's Time to Go to Sleep

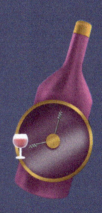

WRITTEN BY
Erin Eva Benevoli

ILLUSTRATED BY
Jessica Corbett

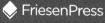

One Printers Way
Altona, MB R0G 0B0
Canada

www.friesenpress.com

Copyright © 2022 Erin Eva Benevoli

First Edition — 2022

All rights reserved.

No part of this publication may be reproduced in any form, or by any means, electronic or mechanical, including photocopying, recording, or any information browsing, storage, or retrieval system, without permission in writing from FriesenPress.

ISBN
978-1-03-911108-0 (Hardcover)
978-1-03-911107-3 (Paperback)
978-1-03-911109-7 (eBook)

1. HUMOR, TOPIC, MARRIAGE & FAMILY

Distributed to the trade by The Ingram Book Company

Dedication

To Owen, for granting me the honour of being your Mama; and to all my nephews who came before you and proved to me that the sleep struggle is real, but with perseverance, laughter, and wine, you will find success.

You've drank your milk,
you've had your bath,
we've read your stories and shared a laugh.
Finally, I say, "It's time to go to sleep!"
You kick and scream,
you yell and cry,
you gaze into my eyes and ask me, "Why?"

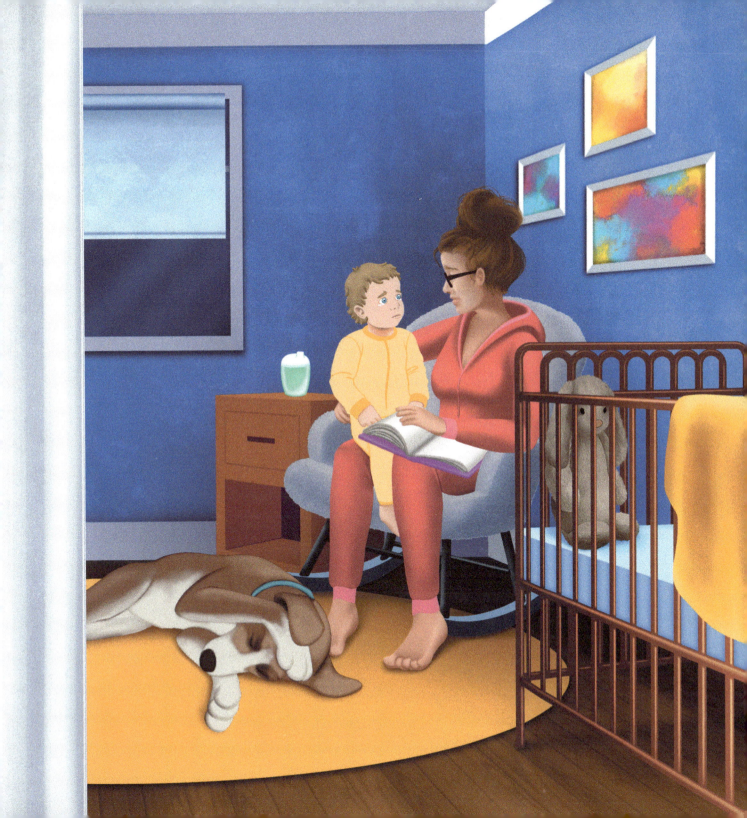

Night after night I hear this query,
I often answer with patience,
but tonight, I'm too weary.
While you put up a fight and sob and weep,
I'll be truthful and explain
Why It's Time to Go to Sleep.

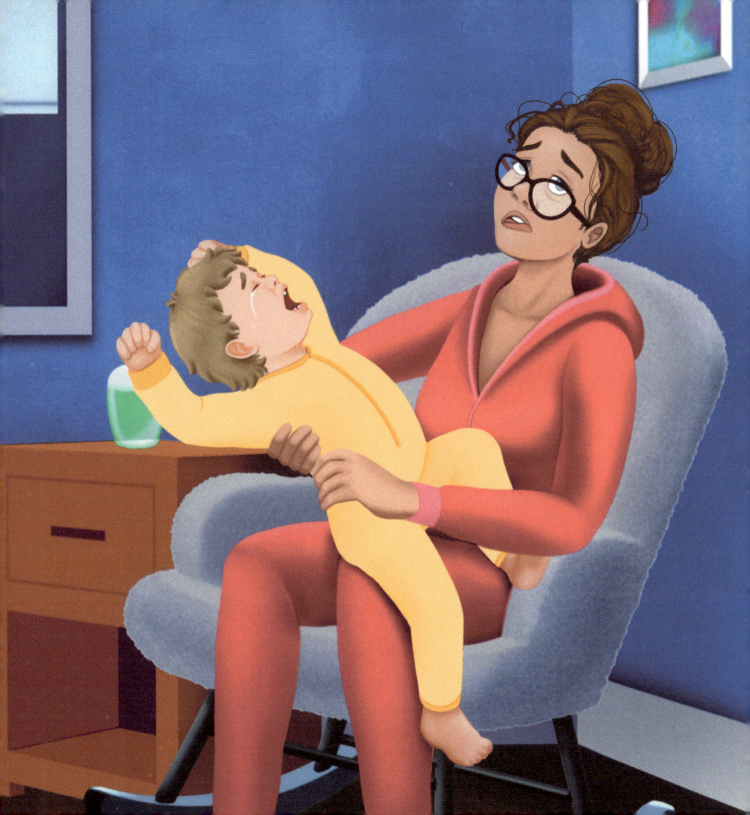

As bedtime nears, tick-tock, tick-tock,
I'm counting down the minutes
until it's wine o'clock.
Now some use this time to kick back and relax,
while others need to tend
to dirty laundry stacks.

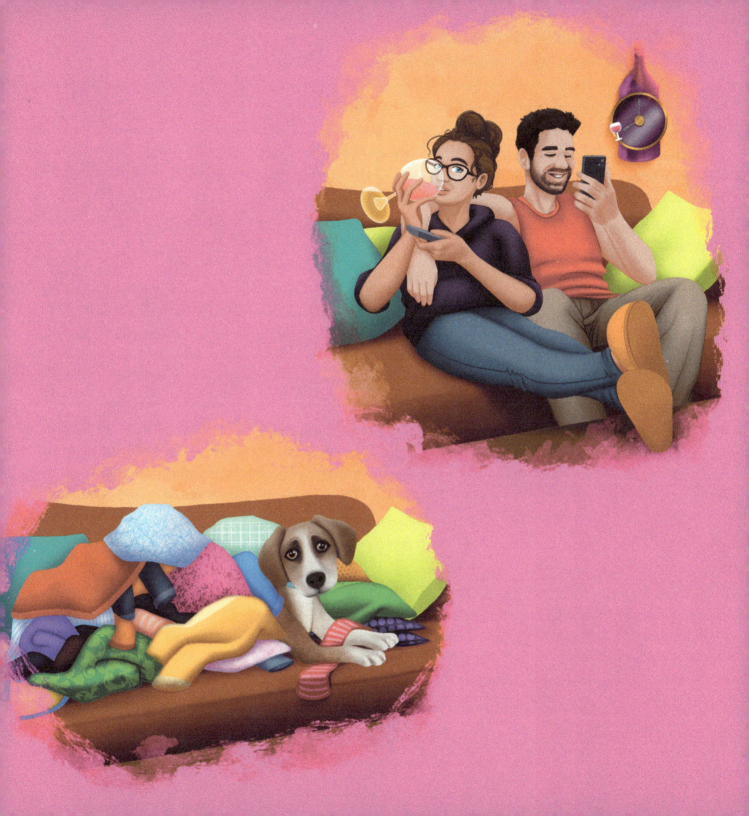

Your parents might use this time to engage
in physical activities
you're not aware of at your age.
Don't be afraid of what noises this may bring,
pretty soon you could be welcoming
a brand new sibling.

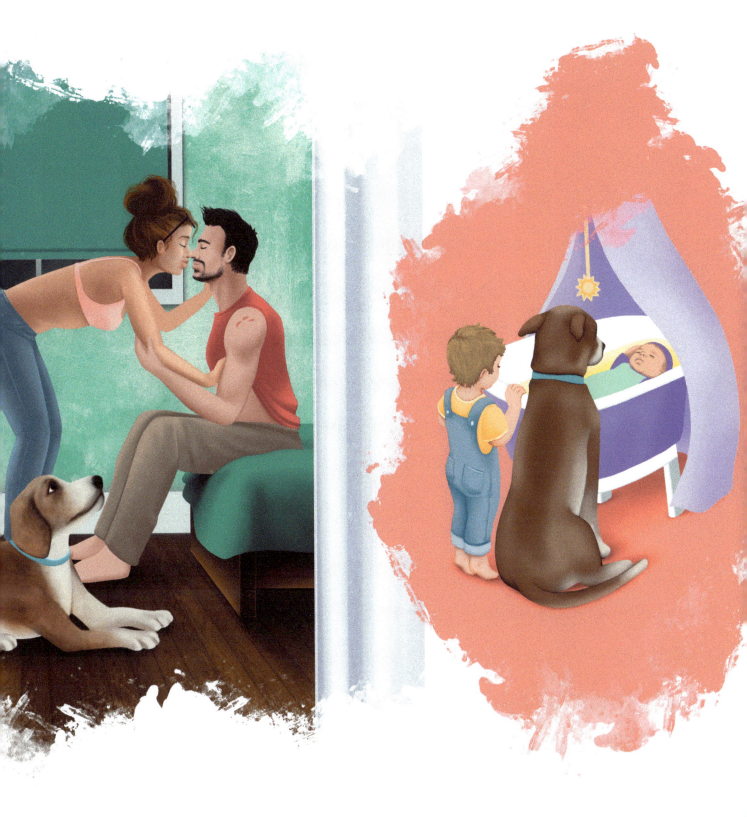

This wine tastes funny,
just off in some way,
maybe because I've yet to brush my teeth today.
I wish I could say that this wasn't the norm,
but after a day tending to you,
I'm in quite the form.

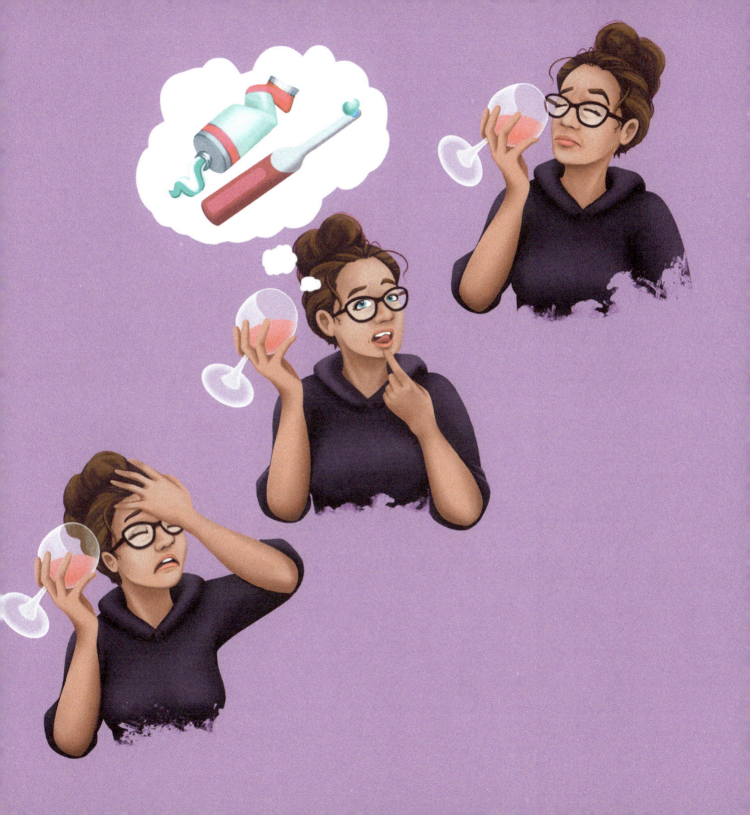

Now I'm scrubbing dishes and picking up blocks and books,
and I'm hanging up clothes
back in the closet on hooks.
I grow more tired as each minute passes,
I retreat to the bathroom
to clean your fingerprints off my glasses.

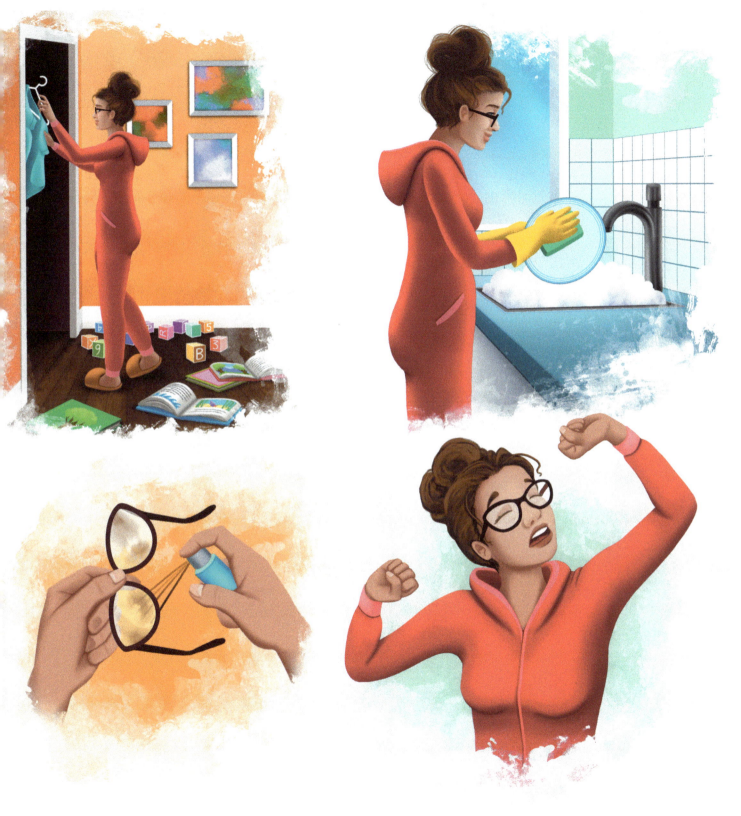

As I brush my teeth and pop a pimple,
I think to myself,
the answer is simple.
Why is it time to go to sleep?
Because I need the energy,
to make the memories we will keep.

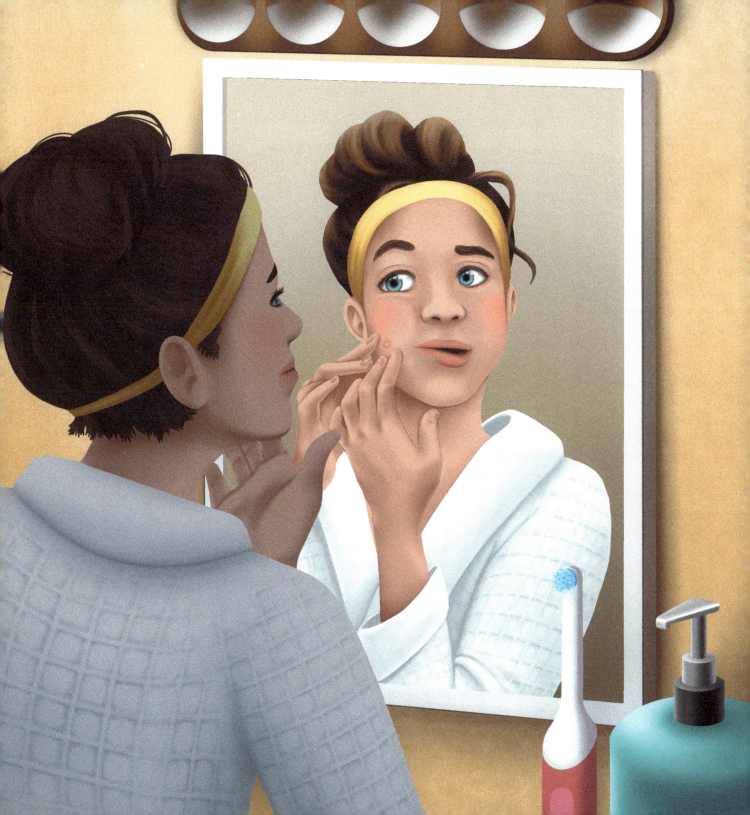

So please, I beg you, we both need our rest,
then we'll wake up tomorrow,
both feeling our BEST!
Don't get me wrong, the best part of my day is with you,
but when you go to sleep,
I get done the things I need to do.

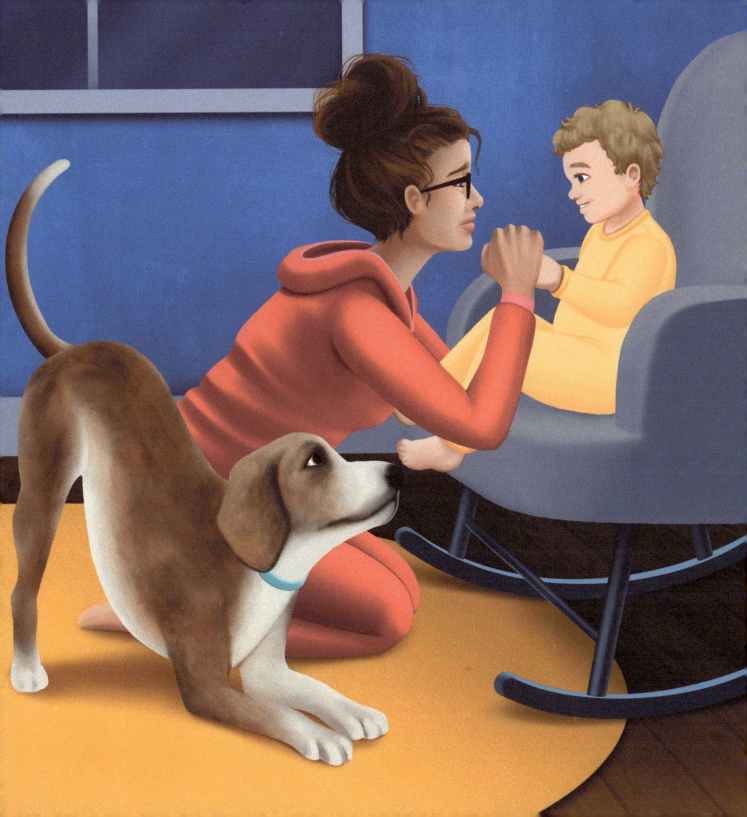

You may not understand and might think I'm wild,
but of this I'm most certain,
I love you, my child.

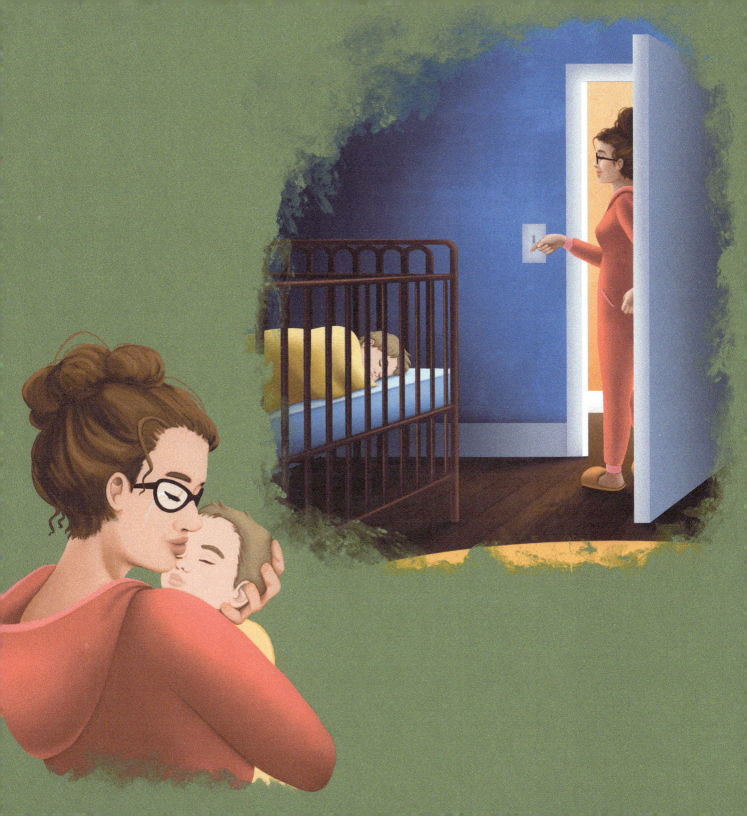

CPSIA information can be obtained
at www.ICGtesting.com
Printed in the USA
BVHW020627150522
637056BV00004B/48

9 781039 111080